EXAMINATION
TECHNIQUES IN
PSYCHIATRY

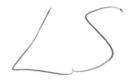

EXAMINATION TECHNIQUES IN PSYCHIATRY

Neil L. Holden
MA, MB, BS, MRCP, MRCPsych
Senior Lecturer and Honorary
Consultant Psychiatrist
Nottingham University

HODDER AND STOUGHTON
LONDON   SYDNEY   AUCKLAND   TORONTO

First published 1987

British Library Cataloguing in Publication Data

Holden, Neil L.
Examination techniques in psychiatry.
1. Psychiatry – Study and teaching –
Great Britain   2. Psychiatry – Examinations
I. Title
616.89'007'1141   RC336

ISBN 0 340 41310 7

Typeset by Rowland Phototypesetting Ltd,
Bury St Edmunds, Suffolk.
Printed in Great Britain for
Hodder and Stoughton Educational,
a division of Hodder and Stoughton Ltd,
Mill Road, Dunton Green, Sevenoaks, Kent TN13 2YD by
Richard Clay Ltd, Bungay, Suffolk

Contents

Foreword

Examinations can be dismal events in the lives of professional men and women. Necessary though they are as yardsticks of competence, it is hard to imagine facing them without anxious concern. Indeed there is a sense in which the utterly relaxed candidate, if he or she exists, might do badly through lack of the extra modicum of arousal, alertness and concentration that everyone needs to give of their best.

Possessing the necessary knowledge and skills is one thing and being in a state of readiness is another. When a candidate is required to meet examiners face-to-face, and when the intrinsic variations and balances of clinical practice are being tested, the distinction may become crucial. Moreover, every clinical discipline has its distinctive character and its particular liabilities to difficulty when tested. Psychiatry is no exception to the general rule.

It follows that there are good reasons why every candidate for a postgraduate qualification in psychiatry should be advised to reflect on the way that knowledge is presented and competence displayed. Dr Holden systematically reviews those matters of technique which should be considered and may be deployed in each part of the examinations. Informed by his substantial experience as a teacher and as a careful observer of the ways in which impending examinations affect the behaviour of candidates, he is a guide to be trusted on every step of the path. No candidate can fail to benefit from attending to what he has to say.

R. H. Cawley

Professor of Psychological Medicine
King's College School of Medicine and
Dentistry and The Institute of Psychiatry

Acknowledgements

I should like to thank Professor R. H. Cawley, Professor G. F. M. Russell, Dr A. E. Farmer, Dr M. Prendergast and other colleagues at The Institute of Psychiatry and Maudsley Hospital for their helpful comments and criticism during the production of this book. I am grateful to the Royal College of Psychiatrists for permission to quote from past examination papers and from examination instructions.

To Margaret and Lucy

Introduction

The main postgraduate examination in Psychiatry in the United Kingdom is the MRCPsych Examination offered by the Royal College of Psychiatrists. However, the College have recently accepted proposals for changes in the MRCPsych, and the transition between the old Examination and the new one will occur between Autumn 1987, when the old Preliminary Test was replaced by the new Part One Examination, and Spring 1992, when the old Membership Examination will be set for the last time.

The old Examination consisted of two parts, the Preliminary Test, which ceased in Spring 1987, and the Membership Examination (which will continue for those who have previously passed the Preliminary Test under the old system). This Membership Examination tests clinical knowledge and the ability to assess and manage patients. It consists of multiple choice questions (MCQs) of sixty stem questions with five parts (2 hours), an essay paper of four questions chosen from seven (3 hours), a clinical examination (30 minutes after seeing a patient for one hour) and an oral examination (15 minutes).

The new MRCPsych Examination also consists of two parts, now known as Part One and Part Two. The Part One Examination does not specifically test basic sciences (which was previously the case with the old Preliminary Test), but concentrates on testing clinical technique and basic clinical knowledge by means of an MCQ of fifty stem questions with five parts (1½ hours) and a clinical examination of 30 minutes (having interviewed the patient unobserved for 50 minutes). The Part Two Examination, starting in Spring 1988, consists of clinical and oral examinations similar to the old Membership Examination, but with the oral examination increased to 30 minutes, together with written papers testing knowledge of basic sciences and clinical psychiatry. These written papers are a single essay (1½ hours), two MCQ papers of fifty stem questions with five parts (90 minutes each) and a paper of twenty short answer questions (90 minutes). Current details of eligibility and exemptions from the new and old examinations can be obtained from the Royal College of Psychiatrists.

The MRCPsych Examination replaced the Diploma in Psychological Medicine (DPM) previously offered by various centres (such as the Conjoint Board in London). However the Diploma in Psychiatry is now offered by the Institue of Psychiatry and is awarded after an examination of similar standard to the current MRCPsych but with a different examination format (without essays) and a different syllabus (with more neurology and more emphasis on overseas' psychiatry). With these differences, the Diploma is aimed to be better suited to the needs and abilities of trainees in psychiatry from overseas. The Diploma in Psychiatry consists of two Parts (A & B), the first examining basic sciences and psychopathology and the second, clinical skills and knowledge. The format of Part A is two 2½ hour short-answer question (SAQ) papers consisting of twenty-five questions each. Part B consists of a written paper (MCQs) and oral in neurology and twenty-five SAQs, twenty-five MCQs, a clinical examination and an oral examination in psychiatry. Changes will occur in the format of this examination in parallel to those for the MRCPsych.

In common with many postgraduate examinations, both the Membership and the Diploma are marked according to the close marking system. This is where the different parts of the examination are marked between a range of 45 and 55. In this scheme 50 is a bare pass, and 49 is a fail. It is felt that this method produces more consistent marking by the independent examiners. However, it is being replaced by a more logical 0 to 10 system in the new examinations.

This booklet is an attempt to help candidates for either of these examinations to improve their examination technique. Many candidates fail, not because of lack of factual knowledge but because they cannot project this knowledge to the examiners. This applies equally to both written and oral examinations and is especially true when the candidate is anxious. Many clinical postgraduate examinations have problems with consistency and reliability, and deficiencies in examination technique leave a candidate vulnerable to failure in these circumstances. The high cost of entering such examinations makes failure an expensive and embarrassing way of gaining experience in examination technique!

The examiners in postgraduate examinations are looking to the candidates to demonstrate that they are ready to move from the clerking role to an executive role. Some use 'rules of thumb' such as 'Would this candidate make a reasonable senior registrar?', or 'Could I leave this candidate in charge of my patients whilst I take a holiday?' As such, the examination leaves the role of testing purely factual information and tests the candidate's ability to apply his or her knowledge in clinical situations. In short, the candidate has to impress the examiners with his or her competence.

This booklet does not, therefore, attempt to increase factual knowledge, or to give example questions. Such information can be found elsewhere. It is purely an attempt to help candidates to make the best of themselves and to try to point out the potential pitfalls in psychiatry examinations.

1

Essays

Essays make up a large part of the old Membership Examination of the Royal College of Psychiatrists, but will play a much lesser role in the new Examination. It has been accepted that factual knowledge can be tested more satisfactorily by methods of examination other than essays. However, one essay paper has been retained in Part Two in order to test the candidate's ability to 'bring together information from a number of different sources' and demonstrate 'the inter-play of numerous intricate variables' in a coherent and balanced fashion. It also tests their ability to use 'accurate, precise and lucid written communications'.

The old Membership Examination essay paper requires four essays to be written in 3 hours from a choice of seven (three in general adult psychiatry and one each in child psychiatry, forensic psychiatry, the psychiatry of mental handicap and psychotherapy). The new Part One has no essay paper, and the new Part Two Examination will have an essay paper in which only one question will need to be answered in 1½ hours from a choice of six questions. The essay will be assessing the skills of synthesising and communicating. Each of the six questions will contain both basic science and clinical components which should be brought together in the answer. Two of the six questions will contain elements of a special clinical subject such as child psychiatry, forensic psychiatry, mental handicap, old-age psychiatry and psychotherapy.

Essays test the candidate's ability to recall information and present it in a comprehensive manner to the examiners. It is stated by the College that

In marking the essay, the examiners will give weight to factual knowledge and to the way the knowledge is presented: credit will be given for ability to formulate ideas, evaluate evidence, communicate clearly and make balanced judgements.

The essays are marked independently by *two* examiners and both sets of marks are given equal weight; thus the examiners have many scripts to read, often with the same titles predominating. Hence it is important that the factual content of the essays should stand out and the structuring should aim to make reading and marking easier.

The timing of the examination

This differs for the Part Two essay paper and that of the old Membership Examination. As the Part Two Examination allows 1½ hours to answer one question out of six it is easy for you to be able to afford time to choose the question carefully and to plan the essay in depth. Also time will be available at the end for you to check spelling and grammar. *It is important, when time is relatively plentiful, not to waste it.* There is no excuse in this examination for producing an untidy effort through speedy writing. You should use the time to make your work structured and presentable and include diagrams and tables where appropriate.

In the old Membership Examination timing is very important as four questions must be answered adequately in 3 hours. It is very easy to fall into the temptation of writing for an excessive amount of time on one or more titles, not leaving enough time for the last question. *This is a dangerous mistake, as four briefly answered questions will get far more marks than three long answers with a fourth answer missing.* Also it is worth remembering that on the older form of the 'close marking' system, an unanswered question will get zero marks, whilst an attempt will at least obtain 45 marks. This would make a big difference to you when averaging of marks occurs. You should use the first 5 minutes of the Membership Examination to read the question paper carefully and to decide which questions to answer. After this, you should use 40 minutes to answer each question, leaving 15 minutes spare for correcting and checking, underlining, and for unforeseen circumstances. It might be that you can use any extra time at the end to add to an answer that is known particularly well. In questions with two parts, it is important that you consider the division of time between the two. *Do not answer one part of a question excessively, even when much is known about it, to the detriment of the rest of the question.*

The choosing of questions

It seems almost too obvious to state the *absolute importance of reading the question paper carefully*, and yet the number of candidates that misread the questions in the excitement of the examination shows that this point cannot be stressed enough.

In the Part Two essay paper there is more time to write and so it is important that you choose the question carefully. If you can answer more than one question from the six, then your choice must be made on the basis of which question you can answer in a comprehensive manner, using the full 90 minutes. Vague questions, where there is no obvious structure, may be best avoided. You should not resort to 'waffling', even when facts are short, and a definite structure should be imposed on the answer. A question that could lend itself to a full and structured answer might be:

Describe what is known about the physiological basis of anxiety. How does this knowledge relate to the pharmacological actions of drugs which are used to treat anxiety?
(Specimen Paper: Working party for the review of the MRCPsych)

Contrast this with a rather vague question such as:

Discuss critically the concept of Insight in Psychiatry.
(Prel. Test, September 1978)

or:

Discuss critically the concept of the therapeutic community.
(Prel. Test, March 1972)

Candidates will find that the old Membership Examination essay paper is much more of a race against time, and as stated above, the examiners are looking for facts, presented in a clear and structured fashion. Therefore it is important for you to choose questions that lend themselves to a definite structure. Avoid vague questions, even when faced with a barren choice. Be wary of questions which invite conjecture and speculation.

An example of a difficult question to answer might be:

> Discuss the aims and techniques of supportive psychotherapy. What are the principal indications for this form of treatment?
>
> (Membership Exam, October 1984)

where fewer facts are required and controversy is present. In contrast consider:

> Outline the indications for the use of ECT. What constitutes good practice in the administration and supervision of this treatment?
>
> (Membership Exam, April 1983)

which relies on a knowledge of clinical practice and current research.

Whatever your choice of questions, *it is often best for you to answer the question with the best potential second rather than first, as the first answer can often be marred by the effects of initial anxiety.*

Writing a synopsis

Structure is needed in all essays, and to be sure that you develop it to its fullest advantage a synopsis (or plan) should be prepared. If you feel that you can write a good essay without a synopsis, then you should consider writing an even better one with a synopsis! The synopsis should be written down legibly on the first half page of the essay and should only be crossed out with one line, if at all. You should start with a short introductory paragraph which might contain a definition of terms, the criteria for the use of a diagnosis, or some historical facts. Finish with a brief but memorable conclusion which should tie up with the introduction or summarise the main arguments. The remaining sections of the synopsis (and essay) can be used to give a structured presentation of the facts and arguments covering the topic.

As well as encouraging clear structure and rational argument, the synopsis allows the examiner to see at a glance how the essay has been planned out. The examiner can see how the essay will unfold when it is read. It may also allow the examiner to credit the candidate, who does not finish through lack of time, with information included within the synopsis. Although you would usually write the synopsis before the essay is begun, it can be added to as the essay proceeds (as writing prompts your memory). Such additions can then be incorporated into the essay in the appropriate places before they are again forgotten.

The form and presentation

Marks are given for the presentation of the essay, but, more importantly, *marks are lost if the examiner cannot find the facts through poor presentation.*

Presentation depends to a certain extent on your handwriting. If bad writing is a problem for you, then you could adopt one or more of the following strategies:

1 Try changing the pen you are using – often a fibre-tip or fountain pen will produce better looking writing than a ball-point pen.
2 Write on alternate lines.
3 Use as many headings, tables and diagrams as you possibly can and print wherever possible.

Poor writing is sometimes a consequence of the slower writer trying to write quickly, sacrificing clarity for speed. If this is the case with you, then a more annotated form should be adopted using headings, subheadings and lists. Underlining key words and facts can markedly improve the presentation of an essay. In general, you should space the work out. However, it is worth pointing out that some examiners would mark down an essay which is seen to be completely in note form, and so a 'happy compromise' must be found.

The style of writing should be professional rather than journalistic. You should avoid political statements and personal idiosyncracy. The aim is to write something akin to a review article as found in an educational journal. If you want to make controversial comments or criticisms, then restrict yourself to those which are attributable to an accepted authority. You should avoid including the detailed case histories of your patients.

The content of the essay

The content of your essay must depend to a large extent on your ability to recall facts. This in turn depends on your ability to remember, and on the amount of revision or learning that you do beforehand. However, just as the structure and presentation of your essay will maximise the effectiveness of the content, the content itself can be maximised by certain strategies.

You must read and consider the questions carefully in order to maximise the effect of the 'cues' that the question contains. Every phrase, statement and qualification in the wording of the question needs to be analysed with regard to what the examiners are asking, and with regard to what can be legitimately included within the answer. For instance, if there is no age stipulated in the question then it might be profitable to extend the scope of the answer into child psychiatry or psychogeriatrics, increasing the information available for the answer. An example of this might be:

> Discuss the concept of predisposition to psychiatric disorders.
> (Prel. Test, March 1977)

where a discussion of developmental child psychiatry or physical and organic factors in the elderly is relevant, but perhaps not obvious at first glance.

Similarly, it is important that you think in terms of the 'syllabus' of the examination. A question such as:

> Discuss current views on the organisation of memory, illustrating your answer with examples from experimental work and clinical disorders.
> (Prel. Test February 1982)

might be looked at in terms of the sciences which are involved. It should be obvious to you that experimental and clinical psychology are important contributors to this question, but in addition there are important elements from neuroanatomy, neurophysiology, biochemistry and neuropharmacology that can be included. Looking further, you can see that it is relevant to include elements of psychoanalytic theory – especially mental mechanisms. Finally, you can draw yet more information from child development and the history of psychiatry.

Similar strategies can be developed for the shorter essays of the old Membership Examination. An example might be:

Outline the major neurological and psychiatric complications of alcoholism. Review the management of delirium tremens.

(Membership Exam, April 1982)

where you might have an initial impression that the examiner wants to know about the overtly organic complications of alcoholism, especially delirium tremens. In fact, it is important for you to cover, comprehensively, all the neurological and psychiatric complications, including the less obvious ones such as alcohol-induced impotence, morbid jealousy and suicide.

Additionally, in a clinically-based question, you can consider the possibility of including information on management, which is often relevant and which is familiar to you from your own clinical practice. For example, in the question:

Discuss the investigation and management of a 58 year old man whose memory is failing.

(Membership Exam, April 1982)

you should be able to write about how you would investigate and manage this patient as if he or she were attending your outpatients' department. Start by covering the taking of an adequate history (especially that of a reliable informant) and mental state examination (with details of the cognitive state examination), stating the significance of the possible findings, and then progress through the relevant basic and more specific tests that are used frequently in clinical practice. Deal with management in the same practical way, all the time bearing in mind the likely differential diagnosis of the patient.

Having said this, *it is important that you restrict your answer to the terms of the question* and do not waste an undue amount of time straying from the point, or giving irrelevant detail.

You can include research findings and publications in essays when relevant, along with references to the authors (possibly with date and journal), if known. You should underline important facts or statements for emphasis and clarity. Discussion of research can be critical but it should be constructive and balanced, and follow the accepted lines of criticism found in the journals. You should define terms that are used and state your sources where relevant and known. The history of psychiatry is important in many subjects and you can include reasonable amounts when relevant to the question.

Revision of essay writing

Most doctors will have little recent experience in essay writing, and you should therefore practise thoroughly beforehand. It is important for you to develop a routine and a style and to try a 'mock' examination under examination conditions to get your timing correct.

Past papers are useful in revision, but those of the last three years are relevant only in that it is unlikely that the same questions will come up again, and there are few examples available for the new Part Two. You can try answering past papers as a trial examination in realistic conditions, or you can answer the questions in an annotated form or as a synopsis. Having read the question, try working out a synopsis, thinking of all the points and facts which are relevant. Those facts which you cannot remember accurately can be looked up afterwards and revised. Even questions which you would not normally attempt in the examination can be answered in this way to give you confidence and to stimulate your memory.

It is foolish to rely on 'question spotting', but it is possible for you to make educated guesses as to which questions are likely to arise at the next examination. The old Membership Examination consists of two sections, the first including the three questions on general psychiatry (one of these often being on psychogeriatrics or alcoholism) and the second consisting of the four questions on child psychiatry, mental handicap, forensic psychiatry and psychotherapy. *Child psychiatry and mental handicap* are relatively small areas to revise to an adequate level, and *it is certain that they will come up*. The mental handicap question usually involves the topics of screening, delivery of services, aetiology or treatments (especially behavioural). The *forensic psychiatry* question often involves aspects of the candidate's *local Mental Health Act, and this should be known in depth* (it is also a favourite question in the Oral Examination).

It is important for you to be familiar with topical areas of research and also the classical papers. The broadest research is often the most useful for you to read, for example, Professor Rutter's work in surveying the Isle of Wight and Camberwell can have widespread application (Rutter *et al.* 1976) (Bibliography p. 46). Recent review articles are extremely useful, such as a review of ECT ('The present status of ECT', R. E. Kendell, *Brit. J. Psychiatry*, 1981, **139**, 265–283). The Royal College of Psychiatrists publication *Contemporary Psychiatry*, with review articles from the *British Journal of Hospital Medicine*, is a very useful source of reference material which can be quoted.

Most of all it is important that you have a genuine broad base of knowledge which will give you tremendous confidence before and during the examination.

2

Multiple Choice Questions (MCQs)

Multiple choice questions (MCQs) have an important and ubi-
quitous role in postgraduate medical examinations and those in
psychiatry are no exception. They form part of both the old and new
MRCPsych Examinations and also form part of the Diploma in
Psychiatry Part B examination. Compared with essays, a different
set of skills is needed to answer them. As shown in Chapter 1, essays
depend on the recalling of facts and the presentation of those facts.
However, in MCQs there is no problem in presentation since the
answer sheets have a uniform format and are marked by computer
and recall is also less of a problem in that most of the information
needed is present in the question. On the other hand, *judgement is
crucial.*

The form of the MCQ

In the old Membership Examination there are sixty stem questions
with five parts (i.e. a total of 300 questions). Each must be answered
by either a 'true', 'false' or 'don't know' response. The response to
one part of a stem does not influence or exclude possible responses
to any of the others (i.e. there may be five true or five false answers
in any stem, or any other combination).

Two hours are available to answer the paper. Answers are
recorded on to a computer marking sheet with the soft lead pencil
provided. *It is important that all sixty stems are answered 'true',
'false' or 'don't know' in each of the 300 spaces* (or 'lozenges'). A
sample answer sheet is sent out to all candidates and it is important
to be familiar with this and the order of questions on it. The

computer marks the sheet by giving 1 mark for each correct answer and subtracting 1 mark for each wrong answer. The 'don't know' response does not affect scoring.

The new style Part One Examination contains a similar style MCQ, but consisting of fifty questions of five items to be answered in 90 minutes, assessing the candidate's knowledge of psychopathology (descriptive and dynamic), methods of clinical assessment and basic clinical psychopharmacology, together with a working knowledge of neuroanatomy, neurophysiology and neuropathology sufficient for understanding the basis of neurological diagnosis. The new Part Two examination has two MCQ papers with the same format as above (each of fifty questions of five items to be answered in 90 minutes), the first devoted to sciences basic to psychiatry and the second to clinical topics.

The Diploma in Psychiatry (Part B) includes an MCQ paper similar in format to the above, but with twenty-five stem questions to be answered in 2½ hours.

The wording of MCQs

This may be difficult for those unfamiliar with this form of examination in that it can appear ambiguous. There is a consensus that the following terms have these implied meanings:

Occurs	makes no statement on frequency (i.e. a recognised occurrence)
Recognised	it has been reported as a feature/association
Characteristic or **Typical**	feature which occurs so often as to be of some diagnostic significance and if it were not present might lead to some doubt being cast on the diagnosis
Essential feature of	must occur to make a diagnosis
Specific or **Pathognomic**	features that occur in the named disease and no other

Can be or **May be**	means that it is recognised (i.e. reported) to occur
Commonly, Frequently, Is likely or **Often**	imply a rate of occurrence greater than 50%
Always or **Never**	suggest that there are no recognised exceptions
Particularly associated	the association is significant in samples with sufficient numbers

You should watch out for universal statements including 'only', 'never', 'exclusively', 'always' and 'invariable'. They are almost always false. You should also be wary of questions that appear to contain double negatives. Extra care is needed in answering them, even when the answer is clearly known. For example:

The following are not necessarily contraindications to ECT:
(*a*) pregnancy during the first treatment
(*b*) acute catatonic excitement
(*c*) patient over the age of 80 years
(*d*) anorexia nervosa
(*e*) clinical picture of depression strongly coloured by hysterical symptoms

In fact, all these statements are true.

Some questions trap by virtue of names which sound alike, e.g. 'catatonia', 'catalepsy', 'cataplexy'. Others bring in names or terms from other areas which 'sound right' even though they are wrong. For example:

The following are correctly paired with the concepts they introduced:
(*a*) Jung: introversion
(*b*) Adler: organ inferiority
(*c*) Eugene Bleuler: dementia praecox
(*d*) Freud: dissociation
(*e*) Janet: conversion

(*a*) and (*b*) are true.
A similar example is:

The following names are associated with specific forms of psychological treatment:

(*a*)   Moreno
(*b*)   Ackerman
(*c*)   Maxwell Jones
(*d*)   Lopez Ibor
(*e*)   John Connolly

(*a*), (*b*) and (*c*) are true.

Techniques and timing

Essentially, *your aim as a candidate should be to score the highest number of marks possible.* There are always rumours as to the number of questions that you have to answer to pass, but the fact is that like most examinations, *in MCQs there is no set pass mark* – it varies retrospectively depending on the standard of the other candidates and the difficulty of the question paper. Also, *it is impossible for you to know with certainty how many questions you have answered correctly: some are bound to be wrong.*

If you answered the answer sheet at random, without the question paper, by the rule of probability your score would be zero. An equal number of right and wrong responses would be chosen. This suggests that you have nothing to gain or lose from guessing answers. However, when answering the MCQ there is, with all candidates, a range of certainty about the correctness of a particular response. This ranges from knowing with absolute conviction to not knowing at all. What varies between candidates is their own perception of their conviction, i.e. their threshold for recognising when they are guessing and when they know for certain.

In short, 'guessing' for some candidates means choosing an answer at random, whilst for others it means having the courage of their convictions to decide on an answer which they almost know for certain. The best advice is that you should obtain a sample MCQ paper and try answering half by 'guessing' (using alternate questions or pages) and half not guessing (using the don't know response frequently). Then it is a simple matter to compare halves to see which technique scores you the higher mark.

Although, on average, nearly 2 minutes is allowed for each

question, time is not usually a problem with the MCQ and it is not unusual for some candidates to leave the examination after an hour. Remember, however, that *if you plan to transfer the answers from the question paper to the answer paper at the end, to leave enough time, and do not forget to do so.* Some candidates will spend time at the end checking their responses. You should concentrate most of all on making sure that all the lozenges (or spaces) are filled on the answer sheet, and in the correct question order. Trying to check that your answers are correct is difficult, as the nature of MCQs is such that the longer you look at a question, the more changes you will make! Usually your initial response to a question will be the best.

Revision for MCQ

It is certainly worth practising with as many sample MCQs as possible. The Royal College of Psychiatrists publishes a selection of old MRCPsych questions, and revision books often contain examples. Examples of past questions are worth spending time on, as some of the questions continue to appear in the examination from time to time. Specimen MCQs for the Part One and Part Two Examinations are published by the Royal College of Psychiatrists.

On the question paper, the MCQs tend to be divided into blocks of questions on particular areas of psychiatry. For instance, the first four questions might be on child psychiatry, the next two on mental impairment, and so on. This helps focusing and concentration, but it also serves to bring home the need for a wide-based knowledge of the whole of psychiatry. *For the MCQ it is better to know a little about a lot.* For instance, those who know no statistics for the Part Two Examination are at a grave disadvantage compared to those who know a few elementary facts (such as the meaning of 'parametric', 'standard deviation', 'mode', 'median' and 'mean') which may allow part of a stem or stems to be answered.

3

Short-Answer Questions (SAQs)

The new Part Two Examination of MRCPsych (from Spring 1988) contains a short-answer question (SAQ) paper, in which twenty SAQs are to be answered in 90 minutes. Half the questions are on basic science and the rest on clinical psychiatry. Specimen questions for this paper have been published by the Royal College of Psychiatrists (Bibliography p. 46).

In the Diploma in Psychiatry there are SAQs in both Parts A and B. Part A consists of two SAQ papers, each with twenty-five questions to be answered in 2½ hours, covering the basic sciences, psychopathology, statistics, social science and epidemiology. Part B has one SAQ paper of twenty-five questions to be answered in 2½ hours on clinical aspects of psychiatry. Each paper is marked independently by two examiners and marks are given on the basis of pass or fail for each of the twenty-five questions. Guideline answers and suggested pass criteria are supplied to the examiners for each question, but they are allowed to use their discretion in marking individual answers.

In answering SAQs, your factual knowledge is obviously important. Less information is given in the format of the question than with MCQs. However, it is still vital that you analyse the question carefully. Often there are a number of requests within one question; for instance:

List the possible causes and describe the features of presenile dementia.

With this question, the request is for 'possible causes' and 'features', and the other important information is the qualification 'presenile'.

It is unwise to concentrate unduly on one request at the expense of the other; keep the lists of causes and features separate and clear, and *do not misread the question*.

As with essays, *you need to answer SAQs in a structured way*, and although some of this structure is suggested by the question, it is important to be logical. You should use a similar technique as in the preparation of a synopsis for an essay. Before the examination you will find it useful to make up lists and systems of classification which will help you to structure your answers. An example of such a scheme is the *medical student's surgical sieve* which can be revived to good effect in the classification of causes of an illness. In brief, this system states that the causes of any syndrome can be:

(a)	*Congenital*	– genetic	– chromosomal defect
		– birth trauma	– intrauterine insult
(b)	*Acquired*	– infective	– metabolic
		– neoplastic	– endocrine
		– degenerative	– toxic
		– traumatic	– inflammatory
		– cardiovascular	– autoimmune
		– nutritional and vitamin deficiency	

An alternative but much briefer system is to *divide causes into those which are primary and secondary*.

Applying such systems to the example question about causes of presenile dementia, it almost answers itself:

Primary causes
Degenerative	– Picks' & Alzheimer type, Huntington's chorea
Infective	– Creutzfeldt–Jakob disease
Cardiovascular	– Arteriosclerotic type

Secondary causes
Infective	– Syphilis
Neoplastic	– Space-occupying lesion
Endocrine	– Hypothyroidism, Addison's disease, hypopituitarism, hypoglycaemia
Autoimmune	– Systemic lupus erythematosus (S.L.E.)
Nutritional	Vitamin B_{12}, B_1, B_6 and folate deficiencies
Traumatic	– Head injury, 'punch-drunk syndrome'
Cardiovascular	– Cerebrovascular accidents, subdural haematoma
Toxic	– Alcoholic dementia, metal toxicity

Metabolic	– Wilson's disease, hepatic and renal failure
Inflammatory	– Multiple sclerosis, cranial arteritis
Degenerative	– Parkinson's disease

You can develop similar schemes to classify features of illness. One way would be to use a previously learned list, such as:

- Neuropathological changes
- Neurological features
- Cognitive features
- Behavioural changes
- Psychiatric syndromes

Alternatively, your routine clinical skills can be adapted to a scheme using the layout of the *mental state examination*. The features can be described according to:

- Appearance and behaviour
- Mood
- Speech
- Content and form of thought
- Perceptual change
- Cognitive change
- Insight

Again, you should find that the answering of the question becomes easier and more complete.

Each question is marked by the examiners according to a specimen answer, with a number of points set as the suggested pass/fail guidelines. *It is therefore important that you try to answer the question as broadly and comprehensively as possible. Remember that each point you give must differ significantly from the others.* The object is not simply to stretch out your list of answers to be as long as possible.

Looking at the question:

List the side-effects of monoamine oxidase inhibitors.

an effort to produce a list of answers might lead you to:

1   Hypertensive reaction with Italian red wine and alcohol in excess.
2   Hypertensive reaction to pickled herrings.
3   Hypertensive reaction to yeast or meat extracts, e.g. Marmite or Bovril.
4   Hypertensive reaction with broad bean pods.
5   Hypertensive reaction with cheese.
6   Hypertensive reaction with banana skins.
7   Interactions with drugs, purchased or prescribed.

Although correct, and seemingly a long list, *this would fail to satisfy the examiner.* A better answer, the same length would be:

1   Hypertensive reactions to tyramine in foods and drinks, e.g. red wines, yeast or meat extracts, cheese pickled herrings (and banana skins and broad bean pods).
2   Hypertensive reactions and other interactions with many drugs (especially sympathomimetics) and excessive alcohol.
3   Dizziness and postural hypotension, and oedema.
4   Anticholinergic effects – dry mouth, blurred vision, constipation and difficulty in micturition.
5   Idiosyncratic reactions – rashes and liver damage.
6   Serotonin-mediated effects, e.g. headache.

In this answer, all the points are different and individually valid.

Similarly, *avoid taking an over-focused view of questions.* Take for example, the question

Name four types of treatment that can be used for agoraphobia and describe briefly your treatment of choice.

This question immediately suggests behavioural psychotherapy as the treatment of choice, but this can restrict the answer. For example, the question could be answered:

Four treatments:
  Systematic desensitisation *in vivo*
  Systematic desensitisation *in vitro*
  Flooding
  Modelling
Treatment of choice:
  Desensitisation *in vivo* using a hierarchy and co-therapist

but a better answer would be:

Four treatments
  Behavioural psychotherapy
  Antidepressants, e.g. tricyclic and MAOI
  Anxiolytics and beta-blockers
  Analytical psychotherapy
Treatment of choice:
  Behavioural psychotherapy with a brief description of the most appropriate strategies known to you.

The following should be noted.

1 It is important that you *do not spend too long on questions that you know well.* No extra marks are awarded for a superb answer as opposed to an adequate one. You should avoid spending longer than the allocated time answering a question, even when you know the subject well.

2 You should make answers *factual, specific and to the point.* You should avoid being too general in your answers; general principles are difficult to credit with the marks.

3 Remember to *use generic names for drugs.* Proprietary names may not be credited with marks.

Finally, books of revision notes such as Bird and Harrison's *Examination Notes in Psychiatry* (Bibliography p. 46) are useful to provide lists of practical and theoretical information in a form very similar to the short answer.

4

The Clinical Examination

Clinical examinations in psychiatry are of the utmost importance for, as well as being extremely anxiety-provoking, they must also be passed to succeed in the overall examination. *Failure in the clinical, for whatever reason, means automatic failure of the whole examination*, in spite of perhaps doing well in other parts. This chapter aims to deal with your preparation for the clinical, and your conduct of the examination. The form and content of the actual assessment is dealt with in Chapter 5.

The old Membership and Part Two MRCPsych Clinical Examinations

Both old and new clinical examinations involve examining a selected patient for 1 hour, followed by a break of 5 minutes before being examined for 30 minutes by two examiners. The examiners will expect the presentation of your assessment, management and prognosis of the patient and are almost certain to ask for the patient to be partly re-interviewed in their presence. The regulations now allow for the possibility that certain patients who cannot give a history themselves, such as those with dementia and adult mental impairment, may be included, together with a suitable informant.

The Part One Clinical Examination

The Part One Clinical Examination tests the basic clinical skills of psychiatric assessment: the ability to relate to the patient, take a history, carry out a mental state examination, and bring the relevant information together as a succinct and accurate assessment. A detailed plan of management is not required. These objectives are in line with the aims of the new Part One examination as a screening procedure in which the candidate must show the ability to exercise knowledge and ability at a fundamental level before progressing further in his training. In this examination the candidate must interview a patient for 50 minutes and then, after presenting his or her findings to the examiners, the candidate interviews the patient for a further 10 minutes in their presence.

The Diploma in Psychiatry Clinical Examination

This is very similar to the above format except that 30 minutes alone are allowed to the candidate between a 1-hour interview with the patient and the 30-minute examination. The candidate is expected to present an assessment of the patient's problem, followed by management and prognosis. The patient will be brought into the examination for some aspect of the interview or examination to be continued.

Preparation for, and conduct of, the Clinical Interview

1 Preparation

You will be wise to have seen 6 to 10 patients previously in examination-like conditions, preparing an assessment on each for presentation to colleagues for criticism. In these, and other interviews with patients, it is important for you to develop particular techniques in directive questioning which are not usually recommended in clinical psychiatry. You must observe strict timekeeping. Try to see patients of different types, and plan in advance the range of questions which you would wish to cover in particular syndromes and problems. You will find it useful to read The Institute of Psychiatry's booklet *Notes on Eliciting and Recording Clinical Information* (Bibliography p. 46), from which you can work out your own lists of questions for use in the examination interview. When you see patients in clinical practice, you can employ this experience usefully by preparing an assessment, management and prognosis for the notes. Also, useful practice can be obtained by adopting the 'assessment' format in your letters to general practitioners.

2   Personal presentation

You should approach the examination in the same way as a job interview in regard to dress and attitudes. You should dress smartly and comfortably. Males would be wise to dress in a dark lounge suit – preferably blue or grey – with a lighter shirt and a sombre tie (or college/club tie). Females should also consider wearing a suit or a formal outfit (avoiding bright colours and patterns). The examiners are looking to the successful candidate to demonstrate his or her competence as a psychiatrist. You must show your ability to extract relevant information from the patient and present it in an orderly fashion, leading on to a planned course of management.

3   Before the examination

It is important that you arrive at the examination centre in good time. Candidates congregate in the waiting room before the examination, and you should not allow this tense situation to undermine your nerves. Some candidates will delight in discussing unanswerable questions or frightening rumours, mainly for the 'benefit' of the anxious.

In the waiting room will be a list of your examiners, and you should make a note of their names. If you do not recognise them, you might ask the other candidates if they know anything of their specialty interests. If you feel that prior knowledge of the examiners will give you confidence or inspiration, then lists of all the examiners are published regularly in the *Bulletin of the Royal College of Psychiatrists*, and it is possible to find out who they are from the *Medical Directory*.

4   Interviewing the patient for the Membership and Part Two Examinations

You will be called from the waiting room by the invigilator, who will introduce you to the patient. The setting will generally be a sideward or an outpatient room, and this room should contain all you need, such as paper and an examination tray. *Ask the invigilator immediately if these are not there.*

Your time allocation of 1 hour should be broken up approximately as follows:

(a) The first 5 minutes

Your first step in the examination should be to put the patient at ease by introducing yourself, shaking hands and explaining what the examination is about. It is worth pointing out to the patient that it is you who is 'on trial' and not them. *This may ensure that the patient is on your side.* You should apologise to the patient that your questioning will be direct and possibly abrupt, but explain that time is limited.

Following this, you should immediately embark upon an intense period of data collection, asking the patient's personal details such as their full name (with spelling, as it is a difficult start with the examiners if there is confusion over the name), age, address and type of accommodation, occupation and place of work, family structure, inpatient or outpatient status, treatment, and what the doctors say is the matter with them. *A list of questions should be prepared beforehand and memorised.*

It is also important to know that the patient is able to answer such basic questions in a rational and appropriate manner. If, at the end of 5 minutes of directive questioning you have not been able to obtain this background information, then you have to suspect that the patient is unable to answer them through illness. In this case, you should check this by immediately entering into the mental state examination, especially the cognitive function testing, before spending further time on the history. Reasons for this difficulty might be poor memory, deafness, speech disorder or severe psychomotor abnormalities. If this is the case, then you can modify your examination accordingly; perhaps an informant might be available on enquiry.

(b) The next 30 minutes

You should use this to cover the history and mental state examination (MSE). The division of time between the two will depend on how complicated each of them is. Much of the MSE will be obtained during your history taking. Obviously, if a patient is demented or severely disturbed in thought process, the history will be markedly curtailed or unreliable, and the MSE must be fastidiously expanded to cover all angles. You should try to spot the 'suggestible patient' whose spontaneous account may well be most revealing and diagnostic.

It is important for you to spend time before the examination thinking about eventualities in the Clinical; you should decide what questions and tests are going to be useful in the MSE, especially in the cognitive function section. Similarly, you need to gather the history in a structured and logical manner, using the direct questioning mentioned above.

Unusually both the history and MSE might be complicated and time consuming. However, you must resist using excess time, as the complicated case will require more thought in the preparation of the assessment.

(c) The next 5 minutes

In some cases it will be necessary for you to do a brief, but full, physical examination (e.g. neuropsychiatric cases). However, the examiners are fully aware of the limitations of time in the examination setting. The patient will probably be fully clothed and there will be no nurse to help undress the patient, so this again will reduce your scope and effectiveness in the physical examination.

To impress the examiners, however, *it is necessary for you to make the point that physical factors need to be ruled out in the diagnosis of psychiatric illness*. You can do this by a brief and selective physical examination. For example, in a patient presenting with an anxiety neurosis, you should check for relevant signs of hyperthyroidism such as the hands (for pulse, warmth, flushing and sweating, tremor), the reflexes, the blood pressure and the neck (for a thyroid swelling and/or bruit). If you are organised, this can be done in a couple of minutes. Similarly, with a patient with cerebrovascular disease you should measure blood pressure, and auscultate for heart murmurs and a carotid bruit (as well as a brief neurological examination). An alcoholic patient might show signs of peripheral neuritis or liver disease (enlarged liver, spider naevi, telangiectasia, liver palms, white nails and 'liver flap'). Where relevant, it is important to examine the optic fundi, the ears, and the scalp (for signs of previous trauma or operations). A full neurological examination would be expected in a case with dementia.

(d) The remaining 20 minutes

Your remaining time with the patient should be spent planning and writing out the assessment (see Chapter 5). There is a temptation to feel embarrassed by the patient's presence, and it is important for you to put both the patient and yourself at ease by explaining what you are doing and asking them to sit quietly or read. *Do not dismiss them from the room* as it is quite likely that you will want to clarify points which occur to you during the writing of your assessment, or ask them questions which you have forgotten to ask previously.

Plan your assessment, management and prognosis, and write it down as you are going to present it to the examiners. It might be that you are able to deliver your assessment without reading it, but it is safer to have the words in front of you in case your mind 'goes blank' or in case the examiners put you out of your stride by interrupting you with questions. *You will find it easier to remember points or sections of your presentation if you have them written down in front of you.*

5   Interviewing the patient for the Part One Examination
Clearly, all of the above advice also applies to the clinical part of the new Part One Examination. One difference is the fact that the allowance of time is reduced to only 50 minutes for interviewing the patient. You should spend the first 40 minutes on your interviewing and examination leaving 10 minutes, which should be long enough for you to prepare your presentation of the assessment (which does not require discussion of the management and prognosis).

6   Interviewing the patient for the Diploma in Psychiatry
More time can be taken over the interview and examination of the patient, as there is time to prepare the assessment, management and prognosis between the interview and examination.

7   Between the interview and examination
In the MRCPsych there is a 5-minute wait between your interview with the patient and meeting the examiners. The patient is removed from the room. *Save this period for finishing touches to your assessment and to compose yourself.* Re-read and rehearse what you have written and are going to say and check that your papers are in the correct order. You should prepare yourself for starting the presentation of your assessment with interest and enthusiasm.

In the Diploma in Psychiatry, a 30-minute wait is allowed to write the assessment on the form provided.

The Membership and Part Two Clinical Examinations

The invigilator will show you in and will often introduce you to the examiners, *but it is worth your remembering their names from the examination list.* You should greet them politely and shake their hands if offered. *Avoid rushing into the room, don't talk too quickly, and remember to smile where it is appropriate.*

You should remember that some examiners will be anxious themselves, especially if this is their first time examining. They may also be tired at the end of a long day of examining candidates. It is important to describe your findings in an enthusiastic and empathic manner so that their interest is maintained, and to attempt to maintain good eye contact with them.

The examination lasts 30 minutes. An approximate breakdown of the time might be 5 minutes for the presentation of the assessment with 5 minutes' discussion of this, followed by 5 minutes for the presentation and discussion of the management, and 3 to 5 minutes on the prognosis, including discussion. Between 5 to 8 minutes will be spent on the further interview with the patient, which the examiners may request at any time, most probably after the assessment or prognosis. The remaining 5 minutes are available for clarification of the case and discussion of related topics.

The preparation of the assessment, management and prognosis is explained in Chapter 5. Usually the examination will commence with the examiner asking you for your presentation of the assessment. However, occasionally the examiners will make more specific requests such as 'Give me the history as you have elicited it from the patient', or 'Tell me the salient points of the history and examination'. Usually, they are simply wanting the assessment, and you should not allow such a request to put you out of your stride. If they want something different from the assessment, then they can always stop the presentation and ask again. If there is doubt, then you can precede the presentation by a statement such as: 'I would like to present my assessment in the usual way'. No written information is asked for by the examiners.

The use of notes for reference is quite acceptable, but try to avoid simply reading out a prepared statement. Stop after about 5 minutes unless you are encouraged to continue by the examiner's response. Watch carefully for these responses as they are a useful clue to the way your presentation is being received.

The patient will be brought into the examination in all cases except when unforeseen circumstances prevent this (such as the patient objecting or showing extreme emotional strain). You will be asked to re-interview the patient to elicit some point of the history or mental state, and should listen carefully to the examiners' instructions. Unless you are told otherwise, you should fetch the patient from the waiting area, and should be very careful to show consideration and kindness to the patient. The candidate should introduce the patient to the examiners (and vice-versa), and see that the patient is comfortably seated before sitting yourself. You should address the patient by name and avoid using terms such as 'dear'. It is important that you use the best possible interviewing technique, not asking too many questions too quickly, or using leading questions. You must listen to the patient's answers and modify questioning accordingly. Before the day of the examination, you should consider what you might be asked to elicit from patients with different diagnoses, and reconsider this after your interview with the patient. During the interview you should consider what approaches might be needed in this history taking, or what questions of mental state you will need to ask. It is common to be asked to elicit a particular point of history, to obtain evidence of hallucinations or thought disorder (remember proverbs, abstract explanations, and tests of association) or to retest the cognitive state (and this should be planned so that it is efficient and impressive). In short, *the examiners will give marks for a systematic arrangement of your questioning of the patient, and will penalise an illogical or disorganised approach.*

The examination time is usually divided equally between the examiners. It is worth remembering that you should try to have good eye contact with both. After discussing the presentations and seeing the patient, the rest of the examination will probably be spent in general discussion of the patient. Sometimes the discussion will become generalised and theoretical, but try to refer back to the patient to illustrate your points. Further information from informants or investigations may be introduced into

the discussion by the examiners, or future situations envisaged.
Some general points are useful on your conduct of the examination:

1   *Do not change your opinions* unless you are presented with new information or realise that you have overlooked some important point.
2   *Do not allow yourself to be led* or brow-beaten by the examiners, as the impression of your clinical confidence will be undermined. A certain amount of banter is acceptable in this context, but *do not argue overtly with the examiners*.
3   *Answer what the examiners ask you initially* – they should not have to ask you repeatedly, and they should not have to drag information out of you.
4   *Do not be defensive:* this does not impress the examiners or gain marks, and repeating the questions while you think of the answer is likely to irritate them.

At the end of the examination you should leave when asked to do so, thanking the examiners.

The Part One Clinical Examination

Again, most of the above advice applies equally to the Clinical Examination in the Part One Examination. This lasts 30 minutes. The candidate will be asked initially to present an assessment of the patient, which should last about 10 minutes. At some point the patient will be brought in for the candidate to re-interview for 10 minutes. Instructions will be given as to what areas should be covered in their questioning. Therefore, *whilst you are initially interviewing the patient, it is important to think of the likely tasks that the examiners might ask you to carry out in the re-interviewing.* You should plan what approach to history taking is best with the patient, and decide how best to demonstrate parts of the mental state efficiently.

The candidate will be assessed on the amount of factual information elicited (including the history, mental state examination and the patient's attitude to his or her illness), on his or her working relationship with the patient, and on his or her behaviour towards the patient during the re-interview. In the latter, they will be evaluating what is asked, how it is asked, and the level of empathy between the candidate and the patient.

The Diploma in Psychiatry Clinical Examination

This follows the same pattern as the Membership Clinical Examination. The advice given therefore applies equally well to this examination.

5

Preparing the Clinical Assessment, Management and Prognosis

In the guidance to candidates for the Membership and Part Two Clinical Examinations, the following is stated:

> The interview with the Examiners will occupy a maximum of thirty minutes. Discussion will generally cover each of the following topics:
>
> (i) *Assessment* – the candidate's overall view of the case, derived from salient features in the history; the findings on examination; the diagnosis and differential diagnosis; the supposed aetiological factors.
> (ii) *Management* – further enquiries and investigations; treatment, short-term and long-term (including the part that would be played by other members of the psychiatric team, and by the family, etc.).
> (iii) *Prognosis* – review of possible outcomes.
>
> The Examiners may raise general clinical or scientific questions stemming from consideration of the particular case. At some stage the candidate is likely to be asked to conduct a brief interview of the patient in the presence of the Examiners.

Similar information is given to candidates for the Diploma in Psychiatry, and some examiners will at times examine for both examinations.

In preparing the presentation of the patient, it should be assumed that the assessment will last about 5 minutes, the management 3 or 4 minutes and the prognosis 2 or 3 minutes. However, it is important to remain flexible, depending on the nature of the patient and the examiners' requests.

In the new Part One Clinical Examination, no discussion of

management and prognosis is required, and the overall level of knowledge needed is more basic. The presentation of this assessment should last up to 10 minutes.

The following is an outline of how you should prepare the assessment, management and prognosis:

1   It is important for you to make the presentation structured, interesting and informative.
2   You should deliver it to the examiners with enthusiasm and fluency.
3   You should be careful not to mould the patient into a textbook case of a particular psychiatric disorder.
4   You should attempt to bring the patient to life as an individual, concentrating on practical considerations and introducing theoretical psychiatric knowledge only when relevant to the particular case.

Assessment, management and prognosis will now be discussed individually: a summary is presented at the end of this chapter (p. 39).

The structure of the assessment

1   Description of the case
This will vary in length depending on how complicated the history is, and on how able and reliable the patient was as an historian; for example a patient with dementia will not be able to give a good account of the illness, and so the history will be shorter (and the mental state examination more detailed to compensate).

(a)   Identification of the patient
You should begin your presentation with an introductory sentence including some of the salient socio-demographic features of the patient, for example: 'Mr Smith is a 43-year-old man, married for 8 years, with two children, who works as a carpenter and lives with his family in a three-bedroomed council house in Streatham'. *It is especially important for you to be enthusiastic and fluent in this introduction, as first impressions are very influential.*

If you have experienced any difficulties in taking a history from the patient, this could be mentioned next. The examiners will then know that they must take this into account for the remainder of the presentation, for example: 'There were major difficulties in taking a history from Mr Smith as his attention was very limited and he was very unforthcoming in response to simple questions'; or 'Mr Smith refused to answer questions on a number of subjects raised during the interview, such as his marriage, or forensic history'. However, you should never feel the need to apologise or protest about such problems as they are a relatively common occurrence. *Such protestations may give the examiners the impression that you are making excuses for your own shortcomings.*

(b)   Relevant background information

This should be included in sufficient detail as to make the presenting symptoms and signs intelligible and to put them in context. You should outline the past psychiatric history (and treatment) and relevant medical history, the family psychiatric history and personal history where present and relevant to the current presenting problem. A short statement of the patient's claimed premorbid personality could appear here.

Two or three sentences could cover this section where it is negative and irrelevant, but such a minimum statement should state that all aspects of history have been elicited and considered, for example 'The patient does not smoke, drink alcohol or abuse drugs, has no previous history of medical or psychiatric illness, and there is no family history of illness. The patient had a normal childhood and schooling with no neurotic traits and good academic ability, and described his premorbid personality as sociable and easy going'.

Some candidates feel happier presenting the background information after the history of the presenting illness. This is simply a matter of choice and is completely acceptable, but *you should remember that some background information is necessary for the examiners to understand the present illness*, and placing the background information at the end of the history may lead to unnecessary repetition or confusion.

(c)   The presenting symptoms

You must be concise, giving a summary of the salient points without irrelevant detail. It is essential that you make the chronology clear, giving a clear account of the development of individual symptoms. You should stick to either dates of events, or the ages at which they occur to the patient. In general, *do not mix dates and ages as this complicates the account.* Mention briefly how the patient's life has been affected by the problems. Obvious events closely related in time to the onset or exacerbation of symptoms should be mentioned here. You can quote verbatim examples of symptoms when illustrating the patient's phenomenology. *Overall, you should be aiming to produce a clear narrative of the patient's current illness.*

(d) The mental state examination

The main findings of the patient's mental state examination should be given using the usual headings (appearance and behaviour; speech; mood; thought content; abnormal beliefs and interpretations of events; abnormal experiences; cognitive state and insight). The amount of detail provided should vary with the case. However, even when negative, all sections of the mental state should be mentioned. For example the minimum statement for a normal mental state examination should be:

> On mental state examination, the patient had a smart and clean appearance and showed no abnormalities in behaviour. Speech was normal; there was no evidence of depression, anxiety or other abnormality of mood, and thought was normal in form and appropriate in content. The patient was preoccupied with . . . (*whatever*). There was no evidence of disorders of perception. On cognitive testing the patient was in clear consciousness and fully orientated. Long-term, short-term memory and immediate recall were all normal and concentration was full. Intelligence was assessed as average and there was good general knowledge. The patient retained insight in that he knew . . . (*whatever*).

Remember that you should not use terms that you cannot define or understand.

(e) Physical examination

You will find that a full physical examination is difficult to do in the time allotted in the clinical assessment. However, it is important that you attempt a brief examination of the salient clinical features, for example examining for signs of liver disease in a patient with alcohol dependence, signs of thyroid disease in a patient with depression or neurosis, and a full neurological examination in a demented patient. You must not carry this out at the expense of a full history and mental state examination, and if time does not allow, a statement to this effect can be made, stating which examinations you would regard as particularly relevant to carry out on the patient.

2   Differential diagnosis

It is often worth stating a descriptive diagnosis, over which there is no doubt, at the beginning of the differential diagnosis, such as: 'This patient gives a clear history of a recurrent depressive disorder of which this is a recurrence'. The differential diagnosis can then concentrate on this focused area (and include endogenous depression, neurotic depression, secondary depression, and other diagnoses that lead on from the evidence). Another example might be: 'This patient is suffering from a paranoid psychosis. The differential diagnosis of this illness is as follows: (schizophrenia, depression, drug-induced psychosis, and so on)'.

Sometimes the diagnosis might be obvious. In this case, state it clearly and think of the *differential diagnosis* within this condition: for example, schizophrenia – a differential between paranoid, hebephrenic and catatonic forms; or dementia – a differential between primary and secondary forms.

Not all diagnoses are mutually exclusive, such as depressive illness with alcohol abuse or obsessional states. With these cases you should proceed to a discussion of which elements can be regarded as primary and which secondary. This is underlined by the fact that patients with abnormal personality or sexual orientation can become ill with a primary mental illness.

List the possible diagnoses in order of preference and for each one you must marshall the evidence for and against. This evidence will usually be drawn from the descriptive psychopathology or the course of the illness. You may wish to introduce more elaborate details of the mental-state examination at this point, such as the content of delusions in differentiating schizophrenia from a depressive psychosis. It is always worth considering, but then probably excluding, the possibility of the condition being secondary to physical or organic causes.

When appropriate, end the discussion with a concluding remark reinforcing your most likely diagnosis or, if you believe that this is impossible at this stage, about the major possibilities.

3 Aetiological factors

In the discussion of aetiology, you can use this section to elaborate on the background information which you presented earlier. However, you should be wary of too much repetition, and should decide during the preparation of your presentation, where to place the bulk of the information. The following scheme, using two fundamental dimensions, can be employed effectively to construct a clear discussion of all the salient factors:

(a) Time
    (i)   Remote events
    (ii)   Intermediate events
    (iii)   Recent events (including precipitants)

(b) Type of factor
    (i)   Physical (including genetic, constitutional, physical illness, drugs, and alcohol)
    (ii)   Psychological (individual psychodynamics and personality)
    (iii)   Socio-cultural (social supports, employment and relationships)

Remote events. You should include genetic constitutional factors, birth trauma, separation from parents, and other important events such as early bereavements and serious childhood illness.

Intermediate events. In this you will be mainly concerned with the patient's personality and the ways in which he or she copes with life. You should discuss the patient's personality and any problems in this area. This may help to bring the case to life. You may consider commenting about the way the patient has coped with factors such as stress, losses, other people, work and the law, and you should question whether there have been ongoing tensions in the patient's life which, when added to by a recent event, have led to his or her decompensation. You must make it clear, however, that as you only have the patient's account, your impression will need to be confirmed by questioning other informants and you should concentrate on objective evidence in your assessment.

Recent events. You should look for precipitating factors associated in time with the onset or exacerbation of symptoms. Be careful before you ascribe causal significance to these and you should inquire whether they may be a consequence rather than a cause of the illness, for instance, losing a job because of depression rather than depression being the result of losing a job. If you consider physical, psychological and social factors, you may find that you are able to weave a plausible narrative, describing how and why the patient became ill at this particular time. You may feel inclined to include *a psychodynamic assessment, but think twice before doing this.* If you decide to go ahead, it is best to avoid jargon and to keep it at a simple level supportable by the facts of the case; *otherwise examiners will not be impressed.* You should remember also to preserve a balance in discussing aetiological factors – *don't concentrate unduly on one* just because it is particularly bizarre or interesting or because you have just read a paper about it.

At this stage you should pause for the examiners to take the opportunity to start discussion. If they do not respond, or indicate what you should do, go on to the management.

The management

1   Investigations

Initially, it is worth mentioning the desirability of obtaining an interview with at least one informant and carrying out a review of previous case notes. You should state who the best informant would be and what information you would be particularly concerned to obtain (for instance an account of the patient's premorbid personality), and also what information you would wish to obtain from the case notes (e.g. a record of courses of treatment and an assurance that medications were prescribed in adequate dosages). It may be important to speak to the GP or the patient's employer, and you should mention this.

  You should then discuss other relevant investigations and be able to justify them all, including psychometry. It is probably unnecessary to list routine investigations unless they are of special importance for the case. You must not forget that there are important sources of information which do not derive from blood, urine and the brain; nursing observations, a social worker's report, and occupational therapy assessments may have a crucial influence on your final diagnostic assessment and management plans. Similarly, a family interview may be useful, as may school reports and employers' references.

2 Treatment

(a) Immediate

Before rushing into the recommendation of drug treatment or psychotherapy, you should think about some preliminary issues. You should consider how easy it was to make a rapport with the patient, and what the likelihood is of forming a therapeutic alliance at this stage. If there is a problem in this area, discuss how you would manage it; for instance, should the patient be an inpatient, outpatient or not a patient at all? It may be relevant to discuss the use of a compulsory order here, or the issues of consent to treatment.

If inpatient care is appropriate for the case you have seen, you should state what contributions to management you would expect from the nursing staff, social workers and occupational therapists and what instructions or advice you would give them concerning the patient's management. For example, the patient might be suicidal, potentially violent or suffering from mania.

In suggesting the prescription of medication, you might mention how you would monitor its effects and levels and how likely it is that the patient would respond. The question of compliance may be relevant, and you could discuss this along with the question of how best to explain the side-effects to the patient.

(b) Long-term

Again, *you should think in terms of physical, psychological and social intervention.* You must consider the questions about medication; its desirability, the compliance, the length of maintenance, the dosage, monitoring effects and side-effects. Consider, also, the factors which might influence medication in the future.

You must discuss the need for, and frequency of, future contact with the patient for follow-up, and the type of psychological help that he or she might need (for instance, supportive psychotherapy, types of formal psychotherapy or behavioural treatments). Discuss the issues of rehabilitation of the patient, outlining your plan in a step-by-step fashion. You can comment on the resources that will be required, and on whether a referral to specialist services will be needed. Without pre-empting the discussion of prognosis, you can discuss practical considerations designed to reduce the risk of relapse, violence or suicide. The 'expressed emotion' studies may deserve a mention in this context.

Not infrequently, relatively 'trivial' measures may make a substantial impact on the patient's quality of life, for example, new spectacles, a hearing aid, or enrolling in an adult literacy class.

Remember not to lose sight of the individual and his particular needs when you are discussing the management. The treatment needs to be tailored to the patient.

The prognosis

Now proceed on to your presentation of the Prognosis. The examiners will stop you if they want to discuss the management at this point.

The commonest error here is to give a prognosis for the illness entity in general rather than for the individual patient with the illness; for example 'the prognosis of schizophrenia depends on . . .' rather than 'the good prognostic features in this patient are . . .'. You should avoid the use of the term 'guarded'. There are a number of elements which determine the prognosis and these should all be covered. You will often recognise a mixture of good and bad prognostic features which you will need to weigh up in arriving at your final judgement.

You must consider the known prognostic features of the illness as they apply to your particular patient. For example, for a patient with schizophrenia, the poor prognostic features might be his family history of schizophrenia and his abnormal premorbid personality, together with the early onset of the illness, whilst good prognostic features might be above average intelligence, the sudden onset in the face of a number of precipitating stresses and the presence of affective disturbance.

A good guideline as to the patient's prognosis is the course of the illness. If someone has shown a recurrent or chronic course, it is unlikely that the future is going to be any different. Conversely, if a patient has only had one or two illnesses with good recovery after each, then the outcome in the future is likely to be brighter. In a similar way, obstacles to recovery, occurring in previous illnesses, are also likely to recur during this illness.

The patient's response to treatment can also be judged from his response to medication and other interventions in the past. Compliance can be judged in the same way, and also from the patient's current co-operation with therapists. Other factors, such as poor memory, low intelligence or lack of social support may also affect compliance. The patient's motivation to get better is obviously crucial, and the relevance of sick role behaviour and secondary gain can be considered in this context.

You must also look at the patient's premorbid adjustment and level of social functioning. Consider whether the patient will be able to return to the same social position and employment as before. A labourer suffering a series of manic illnesses can easily return to his job, but the same cannot be said of the High Court judge or surgeon who has 'disgraced' himself by his actions whilst ill. Social supports are also a very important consideration. The patient might be married, and well supported in a loving relationship, but alternatively if the marriage is disharmonious, then it might be a continued source of stress. The spouse, parents, and other relatives might be greatly involved in caring for the patient, but alternatively, such relationships can be over-involved, critical and a factor in relapse as shown by 'expressed emotion' studies.

You may wish to discuss the availability of *special treatment facilities* for the patient. It may be that such facilities are not available to the patient locally, and the feasibility of travel to other centres considered. You can postulate the influence of the development of new health services or new treatments in the patient's future care.

It may be helpful to divide the prognosis into the short-term and long-term, for instance, the patient may have a good prognosis for recovery from the current episode but be at high risk for relapse in the future.

Summary

The structure of the assessment, management and prognosis is very important and therefore it is summarised below:

Assessment

1   Description of the case
(a)   Identify the patient: Name, age, marital status, occupation, family size, housing.

(b)   Relevant background information. This is given only in sufficient detail to make the present symptoms and signs intelligible and in context. Outline only past psychiatric and relevant medical history, family history of psychiatric illness, and the patient's claimed premorbid personality.

(c)   Presenting symptoms. These should be given with correct terminology and arranged chronologically.

(d)   The mental state examination. This is given in its usual sequence.

(e)   The physical examination.

2   Differential diagnosis
This should be given in order of preference with 'pros and cons'.

3   Aetiology
(a)   Time. Remote, intermediate, and recent precipitative events.

(b)   Type of factor. Physical, psychological, and sociocultural.

Management

Investigation	Social,	By whom?
Immediate treatment plan	psychological	When?
Long-term treatment plan	and	Where?
	biological	What?
	components	

Prognosis
   This illness (short-term)
   Recurrence and the future (long-term)

6

The Oral Examination

Background

In the old MRCPsych Membership Examination, the Oral Examination (or viva voce) consists of a 15-minute interview with two examiners (usually for approximately 7½ minutes each). They are trying to assess the candidate's depth of knowledge and the way he or she thinks (in other words, the structuring of the presentation of facts). They are interested not only in how much candidates know but also how they use their knowledge to answer questions.

The new Part Two Examination (from Spring 1988) has a longer Oral Examination of 30 minutes with two examiners. The candidate will be asked a series of (at least three) patient-management problems (PMPs) which will be prepared in advance by individual examiners. There will be brief questions on clinical topics

> designed not so much to elicit knowledge as to test the soundness and balance of the candidate's clinical reasoning in the assessment and management of patients.

Although candidates who have passed the Preliminary Test under the old regulations will be allowed to sit the Membership Examination under the present regulations till Spring 1992, PMPs are also being used increasingly as the basis for this Oral Examination.

In the Diploma in Psychiatry Part B there are oral examinations in Psychiatry and Neurology. The former lasts 30 minutes and serves partly as an opportunity for the examiners to discuss the casebook submitted by the candidate. The latter is a 15-minute oral with one examiner on neurological topics.

Revision for the Oral Examination

The Oral Examination is particularly daunting, as the candidate meets the examiners face-to-face, and there are few restraints as to what can be asked. It might seem that revision for this purpose is an overwhelming task, but there are ways that it can be approached to make it simpler. You should bring your basic knowledge up to at least the level of a revision book such as *Examination Notes in Psychiatry* (Bibliography p. 46). This will simplify your revision for the weeks before the examinations, and will ensure that you have a global level of knowledge at an acceptable level. There is luck in being asked what you know well, but there are ways of 'spotting' areas which you are likely to be asked about.

You should read a selection of recent articles and papers. It is worth reading the last six months to one year of back numbers of the *British Journal of Psychiatry*, the *British Medical Journal*, the *Lancet* and *Psychological Medicine*. It is also worth looking at the last month or two of the American journals. Sometimes examiners will ask about a specific recent article.

You should arm yourself with detailed knowledge of a few current topics. Also, read carefully a number of well-known review articles. Collections of such reviews can be found in books such as Silverstone and Barraclough's *Contemporary Psychiatry* (see the Bibliography), a compilation of articles from the *British Journal of Hospital Medicine*.

In addition, you should use the days before the examinations to carry out the exercises in classification as described under Short-Answer Questions (see Chapter 3). Plan out classifications for the aetiology and features of psychiatric illnesses, so that you are easily able to structure your answers in the Oral Examination.

Tactics in the Oral Examination

In essence, *you should regard the oral as an exercise in answering as many questions as possible in a limited time*. Each question should be answered correctly and concisely in a well-structured manner. Marks will be given for demonstrating factual knowledge, and for the ability to think in a logical manner. *Time spent in defensive tactics and stalling is therefore wasted* and you are better advised to admit that you don't know than to 'waffle' for minutes without gaining marks. Similarly, repeating the question to gain time to think wastes time, and is likely to irritate the examiners as well.

Before entering the examination, it is worth asking candidates who have just emerged from the examination the questions that they were asked. Some examiners use the same questions, especially PMPs, over and over again. Even if this is not the case, it is unlikely that the examiner's style and technique will change, and this might help you to be forewarned.

You will be undertaking the Oral Examination on the same day as the Clinical Examination and should be dressed smartly and comfortably (as recommended in the section on the Clinical Examination). The examiners should be greeted politely and their hands should be shaken if proferred.

Whilst you are sitting in front of the examiners, it is important that you be aware of your posture thereby avoiding the pitfalls of looking slovenly or agitated. *Do not lean on the examiners' table!* A video-taped mock examination is a useful way for you to obtain an idea of how you appear under examination conditions.

If you do not understand a question you should ask for clarification – do not be deliberately evasive, and answer the questions the examiners have asked in a straightforward and forthcoming manner. You must not be upset about being interrupted when in full flow on the subject – the examiner is almost certainly satisfied with your depth of knowledge and has decided to change areas. Although it is normal for candidates to be led by the examiner, do not allow yourself to change the correct view which you have already stated, in other words, *do not be 'brow-beaten'*. Although it is acceptable to 'banter' with the examiner, *you must not enter into an overt argument.* Similarly you should *never anger or humiliate the examiners*, or try to shout them down in the excitement of the discussion. *Do not make the examiner drag the information out of you* – volunteer it readily, and give the overall impression of being willing to talk.

Many candidates are very apprehensive about the viva voce. *High levels of anxiety can sometimes make the mind lose concentration and 'go blank': If this happens to you, then explain and ask if you can come back to the question.* Most examiners will kindly oblige, and few would appreciate the embarrassed silence whilst you become completely lost in panic. An open and frank approach to the examination can only increase the positive empathy between you and the examiners.

At the end of the examination, thank the examiners and leave calmly.

The content of the Oral Examination

Examiners vary tremendously in their approach. Some will ask a series of short questions and move on to a new subject after each. Some will pick a topic and spend minutes discussing all the aspects. However, the PMP is now actively encouraged by the Royal College of Psychiatrists as the fairest form of question. With the PMP the examiner will give the facts about a hypothetical case for discussion, for example: 'A 55-year-old milkman begins to deliver the wrong number of pints of milk to the doors of his long-standing customers and is eventually referred to you – what might be wrong and how would you manage the case?'

It is worth noting that the facts given, such as the age, are important clues to the answers wanted. The examiners are looking for you to show your ability to assess and manage a clinical problem. In this, the same format for assessment, management and prognosis can be used as was described in Chapter 5. You should start from basics and try to take the examiners through how you would have managed the case if you had seen it in a clinical setting. Start by saying how you would do a full history, mental state and physical, followed by an informant's history and investigations, differential diagnosis and aetiology, and finally discuss management and prognosis.

Some candidates are asked if they have read any papers recently in which they have a particular interest. Similarly, you might be asked if you have any specific research interest, or asked what job you are currently doing. These questions may lead to a discussion of these areas and can and should be prepared for. *Do not feel that you have to be entirely honest:* if you are interested in child psychiatry then the examiners need not be told that you ceased your attachment 8 months ago, and you can still volunteer this as a current interest. Also, if you are asked about research, then this need not be original personal research but an area in which you have a particular depth of knowledge of the literature (perhaps from having presented a Journal Club or similar lecture). However, *if you volunteer a subject, make sure that you do know about it*, as it is particularly unimpressive if you know little about your chosen field.

A further approach by the examiners might be to ask you *what questions you answered in the essay paper.* It is worth remembering that they do not know which questions you answered, nor the marks you obtained, and are simply trying to be kind to you. Do not worry if the examiner does not take you up on any particular topic, but, again, make sure that if you volunteer a subject you know something about it.

Bibliography

ANDERSON, J. A. 1976. *The Multiple Choice Question in Medicine*. London: Pitman.

ANDERSON, J. A. 1982. Answering multiple choice questions. *Hospital Update* **8**: 593–596.

BIRD, D., BIRD, J. & HARRISON, G. 1982. *Psychiatry Revision*. Edinburgh: Churchill Livingstone.

BIRD, J. & HARRISON, G. 1982. *Examination Notes in Psychiatry*. Bristol: Wright PSG.

FARMER, R. 1984. *Self Assessment in Psychiatry*. Oxford: Blackwell Scientific Publications.

GLEW, G. 1981. *Multiple Choice Questions in Psychiatry*. London: Butterworths.

GREENBERG, M., SZMUKLER, G. & TANTUM, D. 1986. *Making Sense of Psychiatric Cases*. Oxford: Oxford University Press.

THE INSTITUTE OF PSYCHIATRY. 1975. *Notes on Eliciting and Recording Clinical Information*. Oxford: Oxford University Press.

MORGAN, H. G. & MORGAN, M. H. 1984. *Aids to Psychiatry*, 2nd ed. Edinburgh: Churchill Livingstone.

ROYAL COLLEGE OF PSYCHIATRISTS. 1985. *Working Party for the Review of the MRCPsych: Report to the Court of Electors*. London: RCP.

RUTTER, M., TIZARD, J., YULE, W., GRAHAM, P. & WHITMORE, K. 1976. Research report: Isle of Wight studies 1964–74. *Psych Med* **6**: 313–332.

SILVERSTONE, T. & BARRACLOUGH, B. 1975. Contemporary psychiatry. *BrJPsych*. Special Publication No. 9.